Mud, Tries and Tantrums

Raising Happy Rugby Players

By Patrick Hickman

Table Of Contents

Introduction

The Joy of Raising Rugby Players

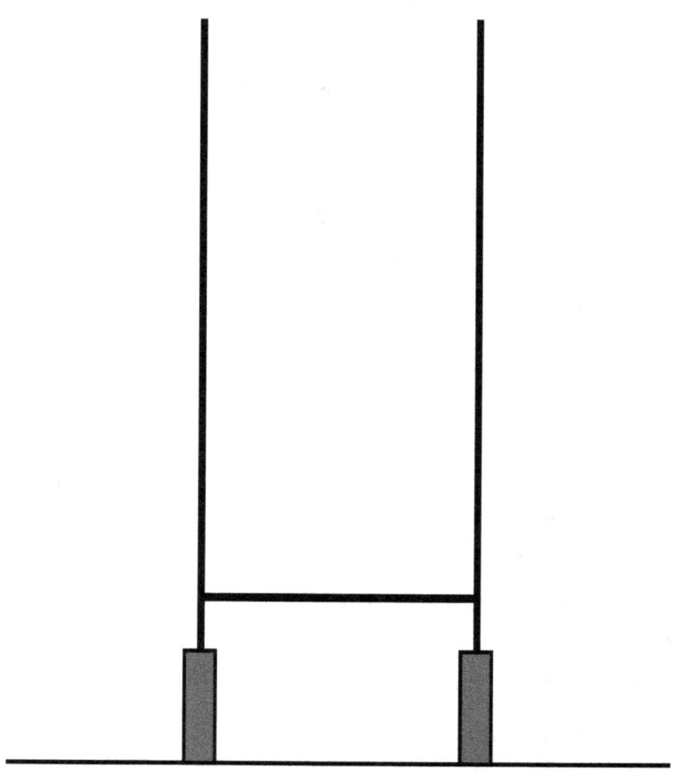

it gave me new respect for those who take the whistle week after week, often under scrutiny from passionate fans like me.

Still, I'm far from a perfect example when it comes to keeping emotions in check. There have been moments when I've let frustrations get the better of me. But the key is recognising these moments and striving to improve. Rugby, after all, is as much about the values it instils – respect, resilience, and camaraderie – as it is about the game itself. As parents, our actions on the sideline set the tone for how our children approach the sport.

In my work as a personal coach, I've seen how our thoughts shape our experiences. It often feels like our emotions – whether joy, frustration, or disappointment – are caused by what's happening "out there". But the truth is, they arise from within, shaped by how we interpret the world. This understanding has been transformative for me, particularly as a rugby parent.

It's this blend of passion, parenting, and perspective that inspired me to write this book. Raising children who love rugby isn't just about teaching them to play or supporting them from the sidelines. It's about helping them navigate the highs and lows with grace, resilience, and an appreciation for the game's deeper values.

Through this book, I hope to share insights and lessons I've learned along the way. By reflecting on key quotes and ideas, I aim to provide tools for parents to support their children – not just as players, but as individuals discovering the joys and challenges of rugby. Together, we can embrace the values of this wonderful game and pass them on to the next generation.

Let's set an example, not of perfection, but of commitment to growth, respect, and love for the sport. Rugby has given us so much; it's our turn to give back by raising players who will carry its spirit forward.

Game plan: how to read this book

This book is designed to be as practical and flexible as the rugby game itself. It's divided into four key sections that mirror the journey of every rugby parent:

1. The Trip to the Game or Training – The moments before the whistle blows, where excitement builds, and emotions can run high.

2. During the Game – The heat of the action, where we learn to navigate the highs, lows, and everything in between.

3. The Trip Home – A time for cooling off, reflecting, and setting the tone for what comes next.

4. Once the Mud Has Dried – A chance to revisit and reflect, allowing the lessons of the game to settle and grow.

You can approach this book in two ways. You may choose to read it sequentially, letting each section build on the last as you move through the full arc of the rugby experience. Alternatively, you can browse through and pick whichever quote resonates most with where you are right now.

Each quote is paired with my reflections and insights, drawn from both rugby and life. After reading each quote, take a moment to reflect yourself. I've included guiding questions to help you dig deeper and connect the ideas to your own experience. This process isn't about finding definitive answers but exploring how the lessons apply to your unique journey.

Above all, remember: we're all a work in progress. None of us have this entirely figured out, and that's perfectly okay. Supporting our rugby-playing children is not about achieving perfection. It's about striving to improve, leading with grace, and passing on values that extend far beyond the pitch.

So, whether you're sitting in the car before kick-off, cheering on the sidelines, or reflecting long after the final whistle, I hope this book serves as a companion to help you navigate the adventure of raising rugby players. Together, let's embrace the journey, mud and all.

Chapter 1

The Journey to the Game

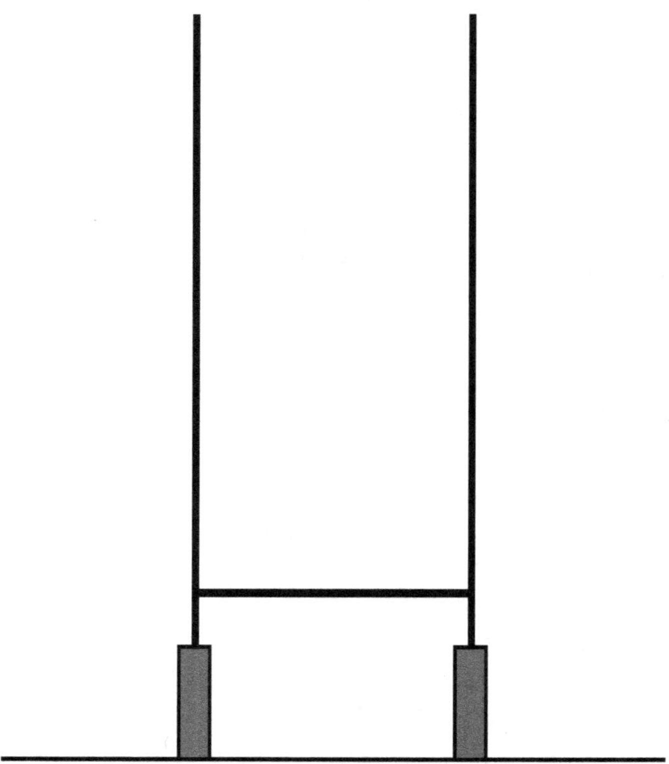

The car ride to a rugby game or training can feel like a match itself. The atmosphere is often charged – perhaps the morning started with a frantic search for a missing gumshield or boots, leaving everyone flustered before even getting in the car. Your young player might be battling nerves, worrying about their performance or an upcoming challenge. As a parent, you could be juggling your own mix of emotions, trying to offer support while managing your own worries. Add in a sibling grumbling about another day spent at the rugby club, or the frustration of being stuck in traffic, and the tension can quickly mount.

These journeys often carry a cocktail of emotions that can set the tone for the day ahead. Arriving calm, focused, and ready to enjoy the experience is the aim – but how can we achieve that when the ride feels like a rollercoaster?

In this chapter, I'll share quotes and the lessons they've taught me about turning these challenging moments into opportunities for connection and composure. Whether it's redirecting nervous energy, embracing the chaos with humour, or finding ways to ease the tension, these insights may help you arrive not just on time, but with the mindset to make the most of the day. Let's explore how these rides can become a chance to support not only your young player, but yourself too.

1. **"It's not what you look at that matters, it's what you see."** – Henry David Thoreau

2. **"Doubt kills more dreams than failure ever will."** – Suzy Kassem

3. **"It's not the load that breaks you down; it's the way you carry it."** – Lou Holtz

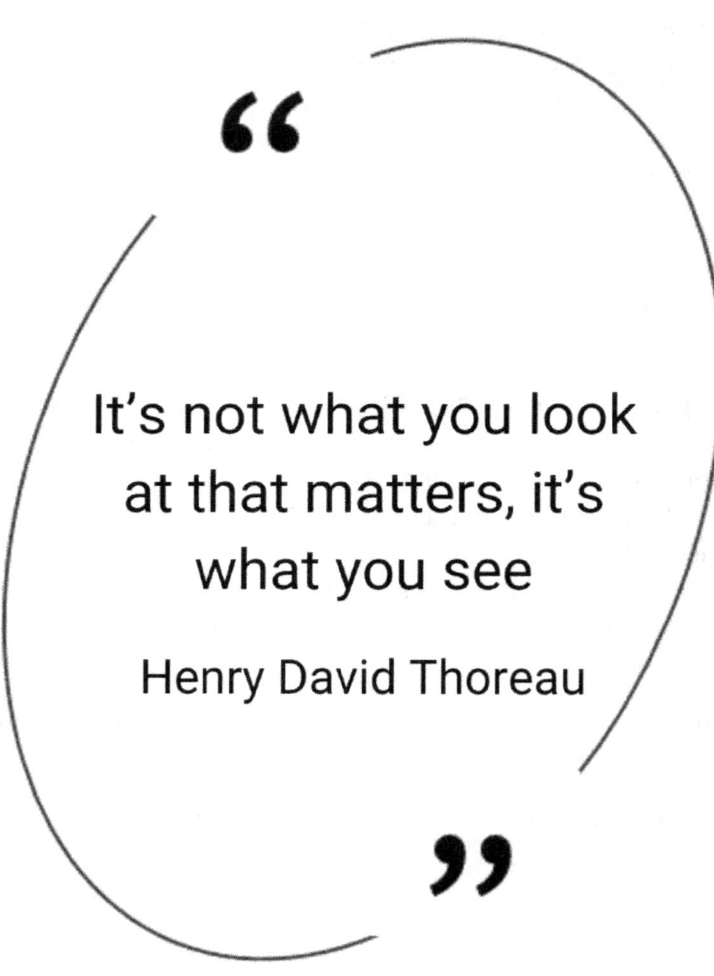

It's not what you look at that matters, it's what you see

Henry David Thoreau

Kick-Off: The Quote in Context

Henry David Thoreau's words, "It's not what you look at that matters, it's what you see," cut straight to the heart of perspective. So often, our experiences are shaped not by the events themselves, but by the lens through which we view them. It's an idea that has been echoed by many thinkers, like Wayne Dyer's observation that "if you change the way you look at things, the things you look at change." These insights remind us that how we interpret life's moments can profoundly impact our well-being and our relationships.

For rugby parents, life often feels like a whirlwind – rushing to practices, ensuring kit is packed, and navigating the logistics of match day. In the midst of this chaos, it's easy to get lost in frustration. But Thoreau's quote challenges us to pause and reconsider: what are we really seeing?

The Breakdown

Thoreau's message is simple but powerful. It's not just about what's in front of us – traffic jams, missing gum shields, or flustered kids. Instead, it's about the meaning we assign to those moments. Are we seeing obstacles or opportunities? Stress or connection?

Our interpretation often dictates how we respond. When we see lateness or traffic as a personal failing, frustration grows. But when we take a step back, we might see a chance to teach resilience or model calm problem-solving. This perspective shift doesn't erase the challenges but changes their impact, allowing us to navigate them with greater grace and purpose.

Reflections from Experience

I've lost count of the times I've had to hunt for a gum shield or a water bottle at the last minute before heading to the rugby club. Tempers flare, voices rise, and the drive to practice sometimes starts with a tense silence or a heated exchange. It's not my proudest parenting moment, but it's real.

Then there are the moments when I manage to pause, breathe, and remind myself what really matters. The rugby kit is secondary to the joy of seeing my girls play and the camaraderie of the rugby community. On those days, even if we're late or hit traffic, the journey feels lighter. It's a choice to focus on the bigger picture instead of getting bogged down by the small frustrations.

Of course, I don't always get it right. Sometimes, the stress wins out. But those moments of clarity, when I manage to shift my perspective, make all the difference.

Stories from the Sidelines

Thoreau's wisdom offers a practical lesson: our reactions are within our control. When the pressure is on – whether it's a missing piece of kit or unexpected traffic – how we choose to frame the situation can transform the experience.

Instead of seeing lateness as a failure, we can treat it as an opportunity to practice patience. Instead of blaming traffic for a rushed morning, we can use the drive to reconnect. It's about reclaiming those moments and choosing how we want to show up.

One strategy that's worked for me is to prepare a mental checklist before we leave for rugby practice. It's a small thing, but it helps me stay calm and focused. Another is to reframe challenges as part of the adventure – after all, rugby itself is a game of adapting to unexpected twists and turns.

Half-Time Huddle

1. How do you usually interpret moments of stress or frustration during your rugby-parenting journey?

2. Can you recall a recent situation where shifting your perspective might have helped?

3. What strategies could you try to approach challenges with more patience and positivity?

4. How do you want your children to see you responding to life's curveballs?

Full-Time Whistle

Thoreau's insight is more than a philosophical musing – it's a call to action. As rugby parents, we face countless moments where our perspective shapes the outcome. By choosing to see challenges as opportunities and frustrations as fleeting, we can create a more positive experience for ourselves and our children.

The next time the gum shield goes missing or traffic builds, remember: it's not what you look at that matters, but what you see. Choose to see the bigger picture and let that guide you through the chaos. After all, the rugby journey is as much about what happens off the pitch as it is about the game itself.

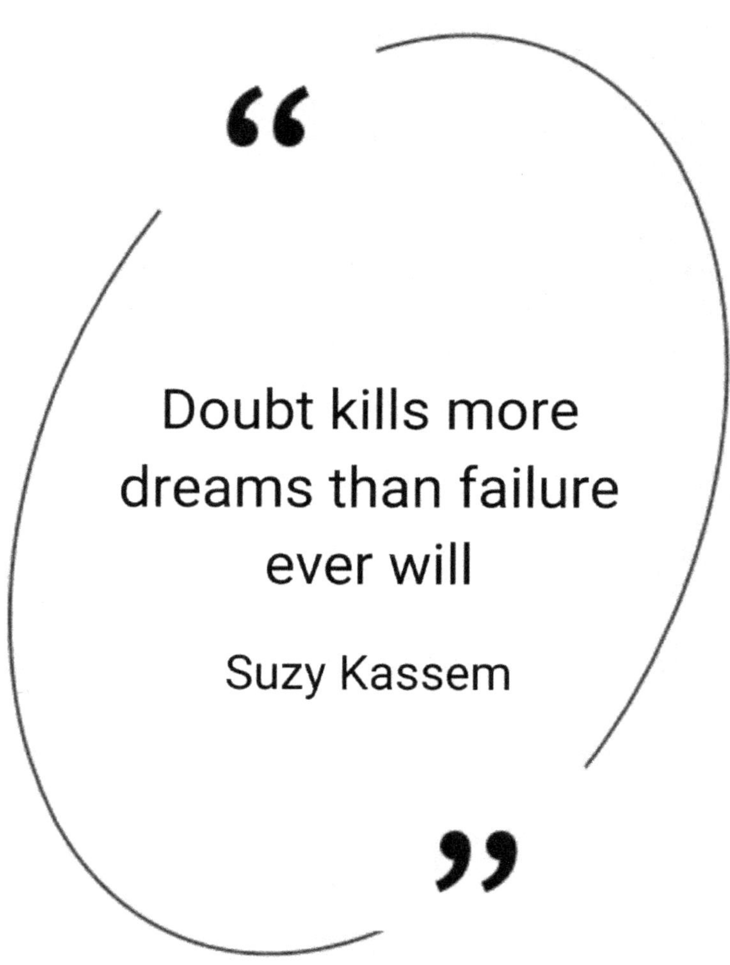

"

Doubt kills more
dreams than failure
ever will

Suzy Kassem

"

Kick-Off: The Quote in Context

"Doubt kills more dreams than failure ever will." Suzy Kassem's words hold a mirror to the hidden barrier many of us face: self-doubt. It's not the act of failing that holds us back but the fear of trying in the first place. This resonates deeply, especially in the world of rugby, where both parents and children face moments of uncertainty.

For rugby parents, pre-match jitters aren't exclusive to the players. Whether it's watching our kids prepare for a match or helping them navigate their nerves, doubt often creeps in. Are they ready? Are we supporting them in the best way? Kassem's quote reminds us to challenge those doubts, reframe them, and embrace effort over perfection.

The Breakdown

Doubt is a silent dream-stealer. Unlike failure, which provides lessons and growth, doubt keeps us from even stepping onto the pitch. It convinces us that we aren't capable, that we'll fall short, or that the risk isn't worth it.

For young rugby players, doubt might look like hesitating to pass the ball or fearing they'll let the team down. For parents, it might manifest as worrying about how best to support their children. Yet, doubt only has as much power as we allow it. When we reframe doubt as a natural part of growth and remind ourselves that effort is what truly counts, we begin to break its hold.

Reflections from Experience

 Match days in our household often come with a flurry of emotions. My daughters approach every game with passion, no matter the stakes, and with that passion sometimes comes nerves. It's a mix of excitement and trepidation. Are they worried about letting their team down? Are they afraid of making a mistake?

We talk about how nerves and excitement are two sides of the same coin. Reframing their pre-match jitters helps them channel that energy into focus and determination. I remind them that what truly matters is giving their best effort. Success isn't about flawless execution but about walking off the pitch knowing they gave it everything they had.

As a parent, I've also faced moments of doubt. Am I saying the right thing? Am I helping or adding pressure? I've found that reflecting on Kassem's wisdom before the journey helps me stay grounded. When I approach the day with a positive mindset, I'm better able to support my girls and encourage them to tackle their own doubts head-on.

Stories from the Sidelines

In practical terms, combating doubt starts with small but meaningful actions. For players, it might be as simple as focusing on one positive intention for the match – whether it's to play with heart, communicate effectively, or tackle with confidence. For parents, it's about creating a supportive environment that prioritises effort over outcome.

One approach we've used is discussing what "success" looks like before the match. It's not about scoring the winning try but about showing courage, working hard, and supporting the team. This perspective takes the pressure off and helps redirect their focus from fear of failure to a celebration of effort.

We've also adopted a simple mantra: "Always do your best." It's a reminder that success is defined by effort, not perfection. When my daughters step off the pitch knowing they've given everything, there's no room for regret – only pride in their growth.

Half-Time Huddle

1. What doubts do you or your children face most often on match days?

2. How can you help reframe nerves or anxiety into something positive?

3. What messages do you want to convey about effort versus outcome?

4. How do you personally approach situations where doubt could hold you back?

Full-Time Whistle

Suzy Kassem's words are a powerful call to action: don't let doubt rob you of opportunities to grow and shine. For rugby parents and players alike, the journey isn't about being perfect or fearless. It's about showing up, embracing the nerves, and giving your best effort.

The next time you or your child faces a moment of doubt, remember this: failure is a step toward growth, but doubt only keeps us standing still. Always do your best, reframe the fear, and take to the pitch – whether literally or figuratively – knowing you've already won by simply trying.

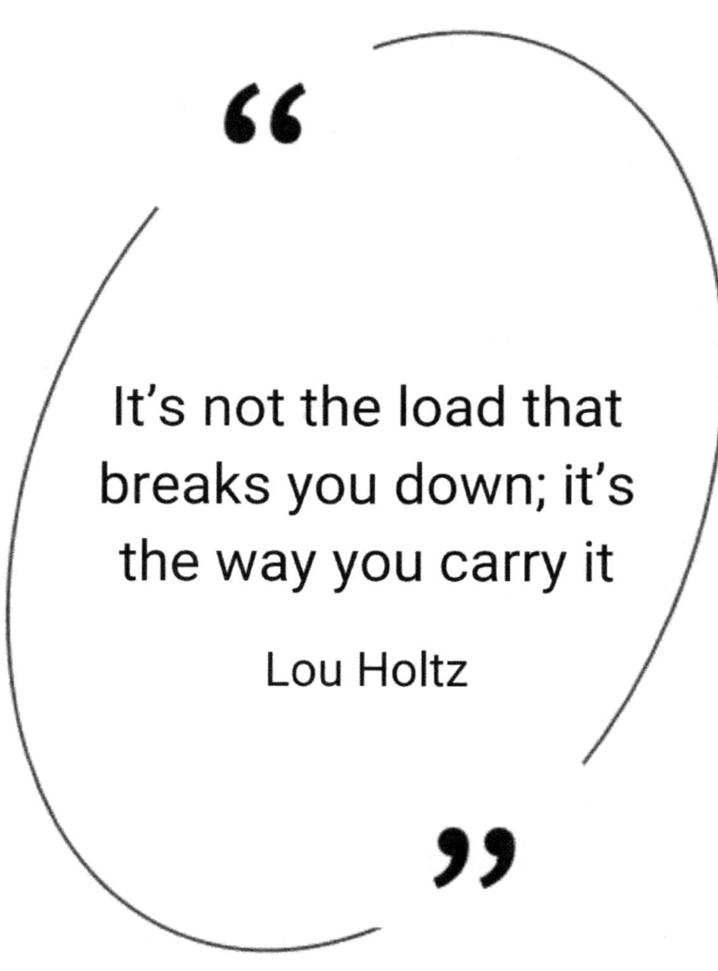It's not the load that breaks you down; it's the way you carry it

Lou Holtz

Kick-Off: The Quote in Context

"It's not the load that breaks you down; it's the way you carry it." Lou Holtz's wisdom resonates far beyond sport, speaking to how we approach challenges. For rugby parents, it's a reminder that the pressures of match day, pre-game nerves, and the whirlwind of emotions are part of the journey. What matters is how we handle these experiences – for ourselves and our children.

Pre-game nerves are common, not only for players but also for the parents in the stands. The difference lies in how we choose to carry those emotions. Do we allow them to weigh us down, or do we find a way to channel that energy positively?

The Breakdown

Nervousness before a game is as much a part of rugby as the mud on the pitch. Even the greats, like Jonny Wilkinson, have openly admitted to battling pre-game anxiety, reminding us that no one is immune.

When my daughters started experiencing these same nerves, my initial approach was to reassure them. I'd say things like, "Don't worry," or "Everyone feels the same." Instead of easing their anxiety, these words often seemed to amplify it, leaving them more on edge.

The truth is nervous energy isn't something to dismiss or ignore. It's a signal that something meaningful is about to happen. Rather than fighting it, the key is to reframe it. Nervousness and excitement are closely linked – it's all about perspective.

Reflections from Experience

I can vividly recall my own pre-competition nerves from when I used to race BMX. Before a big meet, I'd feel the familiar knot in my stomach, a blend of anticipation and fear. Over time, I discovered that having a pre-race routine helped me manage those feelings. Cleaning my bike and organising my kit well in advance became my way of preparing, both mentally and physically.

By the time I got to the race, my mind was clear. I wasn't dwelling on my opponents or obsessing over the outcome. I was in the moment, fully present and ready to perform. This "in the zone" mindset often led to my best performances.

When I think about my daughters, I realise that helping them develop their own routine can have the same effect. It's not about mirroring what worked for me but finding what resonates with them – whether it's a mantra, a playlist, or a simple pre-game ritual.

Stories from the Sidelines

Pre-game routines are personal. For some kids, it might be a specific chant or mantra that helps redirect nervous energy. Others might find comfort in physical activities like stretching or practising skills. The method doesn't matter as much as the result: a focus that helps shift nerves into a game-ready mindset.

In our household, we've experimented with various approaches. One strategy that worked well for one of my daughters was taking a few minutes to visualise the game ahead – not the outcome, but the process. She imagines running with the ball, passing to her teammates, and tackling with confidence. This exercise helps her feel prepared and in control.

Another helpful tactic is making the morning before the game as smooth as possible. One of my other daughters likes to organize her kit the night before and ensure everything is ready. This helps to eliminate unnecessary stress. It's amazing how these small steps can have such a significant impact.

Half-Time Huddle

1. How does your child typically respond to pre-game nerves?

2. Have you noticed any routines or rituals that help them feel more prepared?

3. What role can you play in creating a calm and supportive environment on match day?

4. How do you personally handle pressure, and what lessons can you share with your child?

Full-Time Whistle

Lou Holtz's quote is a powerful reminder that it's not the challenges themselves that overwhelm us but how we approach them. As rugby parents, our role is to guide our children in finding their own ways to carry the emotional load of sport. Whether it's through a pre-game ritual, positive reframing, or simply being present, we can help them navigate these moments with confidence. When the nerves strike – whether in the car on the way to the game or in the moments before kick-off – remember this: it's all about perspective. With the right mindset and preparation, those nerves can transform from a burden into a source of strength, helping your child step onto the pitch ready to give their best.

Chapter 2

During the Game

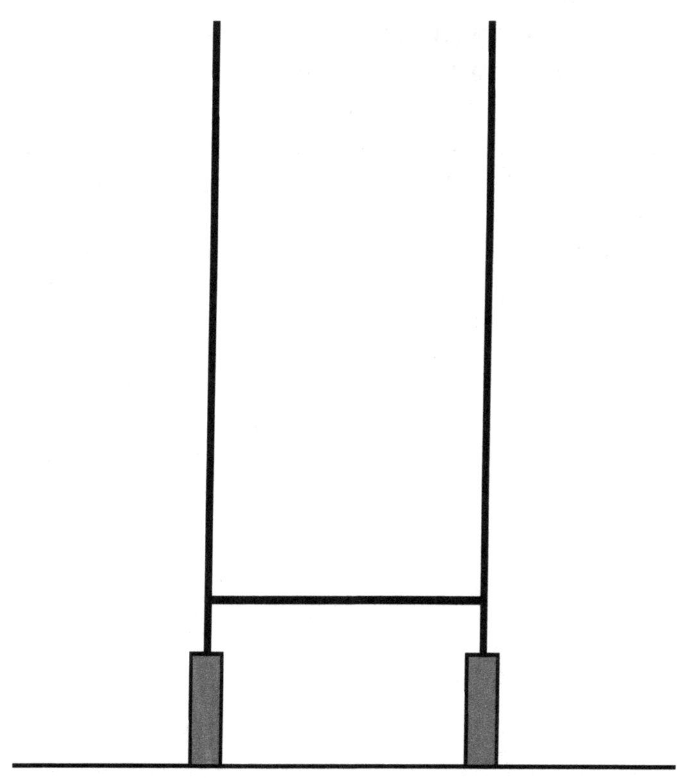

Standing on the touchline, we are more than just spectators – we are participants in the energy of the game. Every cheer, groan, or muttered comment contributes to the atmosphere surrounding the pitch. It's easy to get swept up in the intensity, whether it's reacting to a referee's decision that didn't go our way, responding to an opponent's aggressive play, or even engaging with the shouts of other parents.

I'll admit, I've not always been the best role model. There have been times when my frustration got the better of me, and I let emotions take the lead. Those moments left me reflecting on the example I was setting for my child and their teammates. It's one of the reasons I decided to write this book – because I know the touchline can bring out both the best and the worst in us, and I've learned (sometimes the hard way) that how we act matters.

Our behaviour has a direct impact on our young players. Whether we're shouting encouragement or instructions, expressing anger at a decision, or simply getting too caught up in the outcome of the game, they feel it. And while our intentions are always good – wanting to support, protect, or motivate – we need to consider how our actions come across to the person who matters most: the child on the pitch.

In this chapter, we'll explore how we, as parents, can be the best kind of supporters. We'll reflect on ways to stay composed, focus on encouragement, and create an environment where our young players feel safe, confident, and excited to play. Let's consider how the choices we make on the touchline can positively shape their experience of the game.

1. **"Sometimes the most important thing in a whole day is the rest we take between two deep breaths."** – Etty Hillesum

2. **"Correction does much, but encouragement does more."** – Johann Wolfgang von Goethe

3. **"I've failed over and over and over again in my life. And that is why I succeed."** – Michael Jordan

Sometimes the most important thing in a whole day is the rest we take between two deep breaths

Etty Hillesum

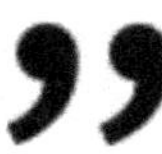

Kick-Off: The Quote in Context

Rugby is more than a game; it's an emotional rollercoaster. For those of us on the sidelines, watching our children play can be as intense as any match they're in. We feel their highs and lows, the excitement of a well-executed play, and the frustration when things don't go their way – or ours. Etty Hillesum's words remind us of the power of pausing, taking a breath, and grounding ourselves.

"Sometimes the most important thing in a whole day is the rest we take between two deep breaths." This quote speaks directly to the challenges of maintaining balance in emotionally charged moments, such as when we feel tempted to shout at a missed call or a mistake on the pitch.

The Breakdown

Rugby matches have a way of stirring strong emotions in parents. Whether it's seeing our children struggle, a referee's missed call, or a team decision that doesn't pan out, we can easily get caught up in the moment. These reactions are natural; they stem from our desire to see our children succeed and stay safe.

But when emotions take over, they can cloud our judgment. Staying calm requires conscious effort, particularly when we're "off guard." The power of a deep breath can't be overstated. It's a simple but effective tool to reset our energy and focus. Those moments of pause create space for us to choose how we respond, rather than reacting instinctively.

Reflections from Experience

I've been there – standing on the sidelines, heart racing, watching a game unfold in a way that challenges my composure. When the referee misses a high tackle, or my daughter drops the ball, I feel the heat of frustration rising. Early on, I struggled to manage those moments. I'd find myself clenching my fists, pacing, or even muttering under my breath.

Over time, I've realised that stepping away, physically and mentally, is often the best course of action. Walking a few steps away from the pitch or even focusing on the rhythm of my breathing can make all the difference.

One thing I've carried over from parenting is the habit of using deep breathing with my daughters. When they're overwhelmed, I get down to their level, encourage them to take a few slow breaths, and sometimes mirror my own breathing for them to follow. It's remarkable how quickly it restores calm – not only for them but for me too.

Stories from the Sidelines

Keeping calm during a match benefits more than just your nerves – it allows you to see the game objectively. When emotions aren't running high, you can appreciate the game for what it is: an opportunity for your child to learn, grow, and enjoy.

Taking a step back also sets a positive example. Rugby is a game built on respect – for teammates, opponents, referees, and coaches. By staying composed, we model the very values we want our children to embrace. It's easier to have productive conversations after the final whistle when you've remained level-headed during the match.

On a practical level, I've found it helpful to prepare myself mentally before a game. I remind myself that mistakes are inevitable, and that players and referees are human. Most importantly, I commit to staying grounded by using my breath as a tool. A few slow, deliberate breaths during tense moments can restore equilibrium and allow me to refocus on the joy of watching my child play.

Half-Time Huddle

1. How do you typically react when emotions rise on the sidelines?

2. What strategies have you tried to manage these moments?

3. How can you model calmness and respect during games, even when tensions run high?

4. What role do you think preparation plays in handling the emotional ups and downs of watching a match?

5. How can you use the lessons from breathing exercises to help your child handle their own moments of stress?

Full-Time Whistle

Etty Hillesum's quote offers a valuable reminder for rugby parents: sometimes, the most important thing we can do is pause and take a breath. Those moments of rest allow us to regain balance, make better decisions, and enjoy the experience of supporting our children.

Rugby isn't just about the game – it's about the lessons it teaches us as parents and players alike. Staying calm, even during high-stakes moments, enables us to appreciate the journey and model the respect and composure we want our children to carry onto the pitch.

So, the next time emotions rise during a match, take a moment. Breathe deeply. Let the pause bring perspective, allowing you to focus on what truly matters: the privilege of watching your child grow through the game we all love.

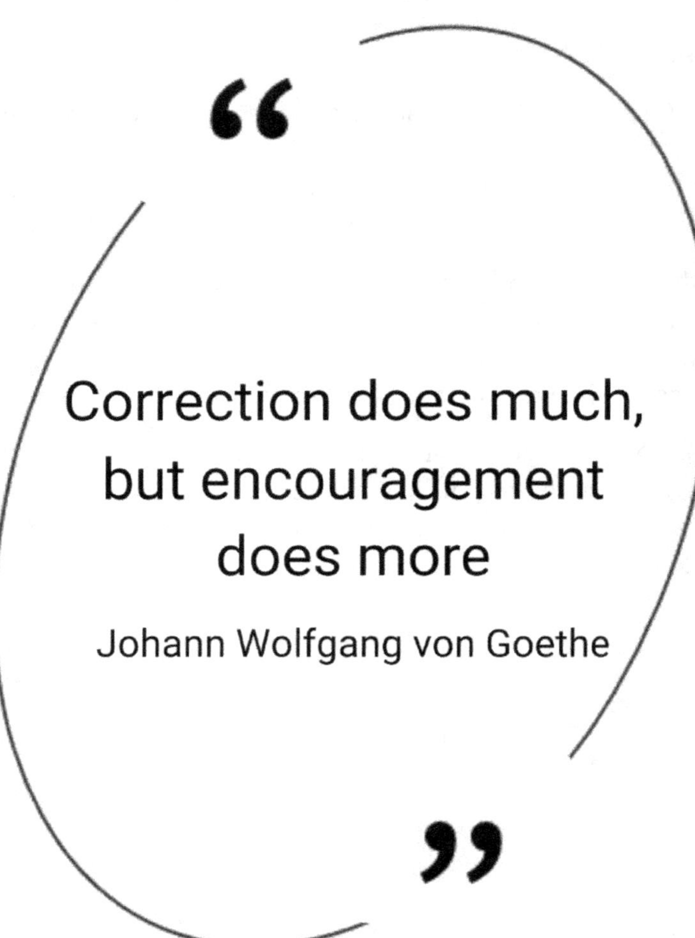

Correction does much,
but encouragement
does more

Johann Wolfgang von Goethe

Kick-Off: The Quote in Context

Rugby is a game of endless movement, where the landscape changes from one second to the next. It's the same with parenting and coaching – no two moments are ever quite the same. Johann Wolfgang von Goethe's quote, "Correction does much, but encouragement does more," reminds us of the power of positive reinforcement, especially when watching our children play.

It's easy to focus on what could be improved. We've all caught ourselves offering advice from the sidelines or pointing out areas for adjustment. But in a sport as dynamic as rugby, players thrive on confidence, and confidence is built through encouragement, not criticism.

The Breakdown

Criticism often stems from a good place. We want to help, to guide, to make sure our children avoid mistakes we think we can foresee. But what we forget is that rugby, like life, is not a rigid set of scenarios to solve with pre-determined answers. It's fluid, unpredictable, and requires the ability to adapt on the fly.

When we focus too much on correction, we can unintentionally stifle our children's ability to explore and experiment. Rugby players, especially young ones, need the freedom to make decisions in the moment. Yes, there will be errors, but those mistakes are where the real learning happens. Encouragement, on the other hand, builds resilience, motivation, and the willingness to keep trying even when things go wrong.

Reflections from Experience

As a coach and parent, I've had to learn this lesson the hard way. I can remember a time when I was more focused on pointing out what my daughters could do differently than cheering them on for what they did well. It didn't take long to notice that this approach often left them frustrated and discouraged.

Over time, I realised that stepping back and letting them figure things out on their own made a huge difference. I began setting boundaries and giving them the freedom to solve problems in their own way. My role shifted from constant instructor to supportive observer.

On the sidelines, I started focusing on encouragement rather than critique. "Great pass!" or "Excellent tackle!" became my go-to phrases, and I could see how those simple words made their faces light up and their confidence grow. It wasn't about ignoring mistakes but choosing not to dwell on them.

Stories from the Sidelines

One of rugby's greatest strengths is its unpredictability. No two matches are the same, and no two moments within a game play out identically. This is why prescriptive advice often falls flat – it doesn't account for the constantly changing context of the game.

Our children need to learn to read these situations for themselves, to make decisions based on what they see in front of them. When we focus on encouragement rather than correction, we empower them to trust their instincts and develop that decision-making ability.

Encouragement isn't about turning a blind eye to improvement. It's about recognising the effort, celebrating progress, and fostering the love of the game. That love is what will keep them coming back, striving to be better, and finding joy in the process.

Half-Time Huddle

1. How do you balance offering guidance with giving your child space to learn independently?

2. Can you recall a time when encouragement helped your child overcome a challenge?

3. What strategies can you use to focus on positive reinforcement
    during games?

4. How might shifting from corrective feedback to encouragement
    change your child's perception of the game?

5. What role does making mistakes play in developing both
    confidence and skill?

Full-Time Whistle

Goethe's words remind us that while correction has its place,
encouragement is what truly inspires growth. As rugby parents, we have
a unique role to play in shaping how our children experience the game.
By choosing to focus on what they're doing well, we can build their
confidence and motivation. This not only helps them enjoy the sport but
also equips them with the resilience and adaptability they'll need both
on and off the pitch.

So, the next time you're standing on the sidelines, remember that your
cheers hold more power than your advice. Let your voice be the one that
lifts them up, giving them the confidence to tackle whatever comes their
way.

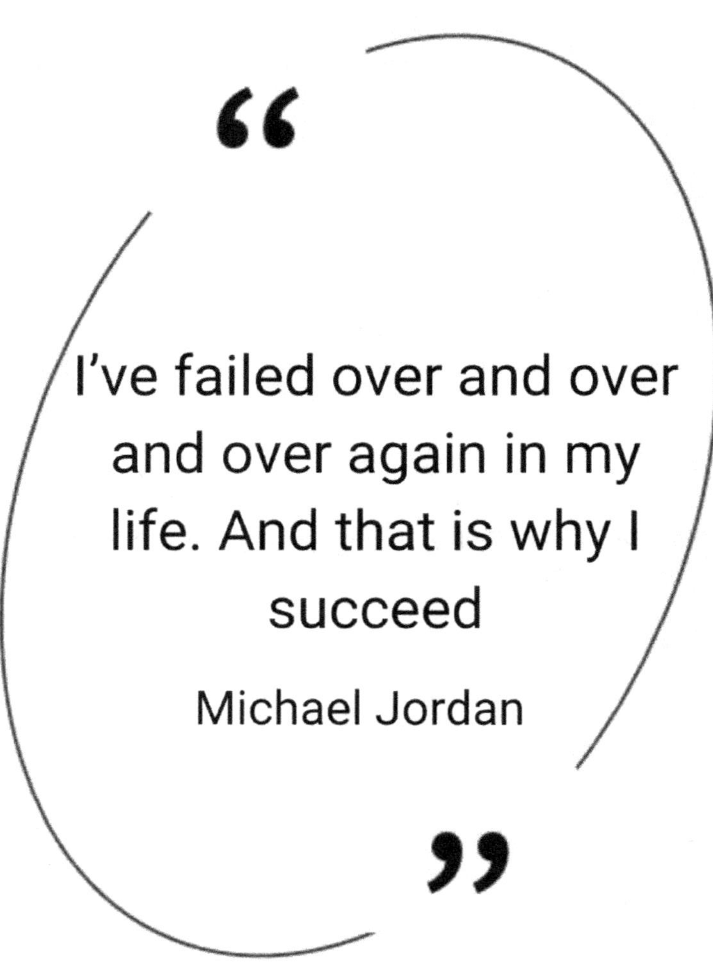

I've failed over and over
and over again in my
life. And that is why I
succeed

Michael Jordan

Kick-Off: The Quote in Context

Michael Jordan's quote hits on a universal truth: success is built on failure. Whether on the court, the pitch, or in life, failure is not the enemy – it's the teacher. For rugby parents, this concept resonates deeply. Watching our children play is a rollercoaster of emotions. We cheer for their triumphs, but witnessing their struggles or mistakes can leave us anxious or frustrated.

However, this quote serves as a powerful reminder that every stumble, dropped pass, or missed tackle is part of the journey. Mistakes are not roadblocks; they're stepping stones to success. By reframing how we view failure, both in sport and in life, we can better support our children in their growth, resilience, and self-confidence.

The Breakdown

One of the biggest hurdles in parenting and coaching young athletes is helping them understand that mistakes are a natural and necessary part of improvement. Many children approach sports with a fear of failing. It's a fear that often stems from the schooling system, where success is measured by getting things right and failure is something to avoid.

But rugby, much like life, doesn't work that way. Rugby is a game of constant adaptation. Decisions are made in split seconds, and no two plays are ever the same. To succeed, players must be willing to experiment, take risks, and learn from the inevitable mistakes.

Michael Jordan's journey embodies this truth. His incredible success wasn't due to avoiding failure but embracing it as part of his growth. The same principle applies to our children. The more they try – and fail – the closer they'll come to finding what works and building their confidence.

Reflections from Experience

As a coach and a parent, I've encountered countless examples of children holding back for fear of making mistakes. I vividly remember one match where a young player hesitated to kick the ball when under pressure on their try line. When they finally did, the timing was off, the kick was wayward, and the opposition gathered it easily and scored. From the sidelines, I could hear the familiar cries of "Don't kick!"

That moment could have shattered the player's confidence, but instead, we turned it into a learning opportunity. We talked about what went wrong – timing, positioning, technique – and how to approach a similar situation in the future. Later in the season, that same player executed a perfect clearing kick under pressure. The pride they felt in that moment was immeasurable, and it stemmed directly from their earlier mistake.

This experience reinforced for me the importance of embracing failure as part of the process. Our children won't grow into skilled and confident players if they're afraid to try. Every missed tackle, misjudged pass, or poorly timed kick is an opportunity to learn and improve.

Stories from the Sidelines

As parents, our role on the sidelines is crucial. By encouraging effort and experimentation, we help our children develop resilience and adaptability. This doesn't mean ignoring mistakes but framing them in a way that fosters growth. Instead of criticising a decision that didn't work out, we can focus on what can be learned.

One of the most valuable lessons rugby can teach is how to assess and adapt. The game moves quickly, requiring players to make decisions in real-time. This is why rigidly prescribing what they should or shouldn't do is unhelpful. Telling a child never to kick or always to pass denies them the opportunity to learn through experience.

The greatest players in the world didn't arrive at their level of skill without countless failed attempts. Think of a young player attempting a high-risk pass that doesn't come off. They've just learned something valuable: how to judge timing, assess spacing, and perhaps when to take a safer option. With time and repetition, those lessons turn into instinct.

As parents, we must also learn to manage our own emotions. It can be difficult to watch our children struggle, but offering encouragement and constructive feedback is far more impactful than sideline criticism. Our

words and actions shape how our children perceive their mistakes –
whether they see them as something to avoid or as essential steps
towards success.

Half-Time Huddle

1. How do you react when your child makes a mistake during a
   game?

2. Are you modelling resilience and a growth mindset in your own
   life?

3. What steps can you take to ensure your child views mistakes as
   learning opportunities rather than failures?

4. How can you reframe a recent challenging moment for your child
   into a positive learning experience?

Full-Time Whistle

Michael Jordan's quote is a call to action for all of us – parents, coaches,
and players alike. It reminds us that failure is not the end of the story; it's
the beginning. Every mistake our children make on the rugby pitch is a
building block for their future success, both in sport and in life.

By embracing failure as part of the process, we allow our children to
explore, adapt, and grow. It's not about shielding them from struggle but
supporting them as they navigate it. Let's cheer them on as they take
risks, make mistakes, and discover their own paths.

With patience, encouragement, and the understanding that failure is a
powerful teacher, we can help our children build the resilience and
confidence they need to succeed – not just on the pitch, but in every
area of their lives.

Chapter 3

The Car Ride Home

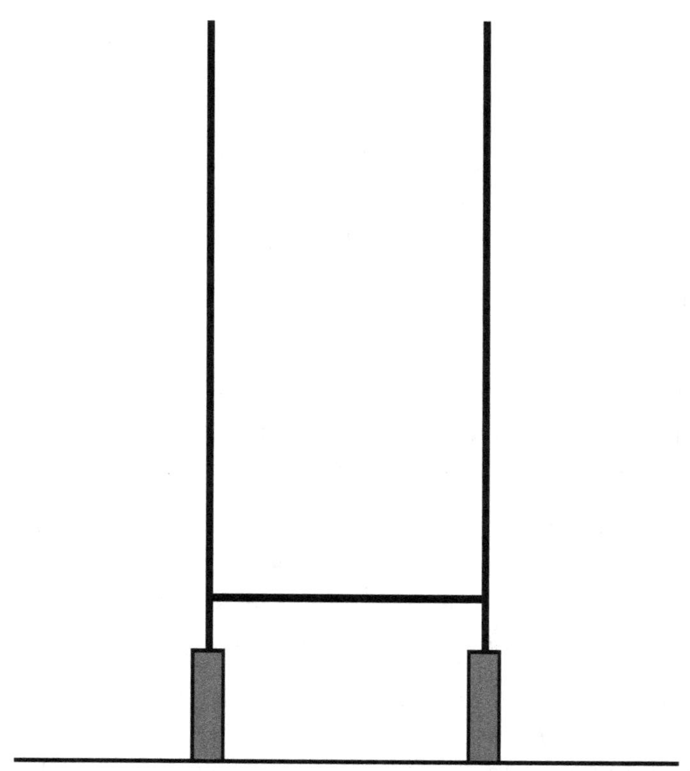

The journey home from a game can be a delicate time. Emotions are still raw – your child might be replaying a missed tackle, a difficult interaction with a teammate, or something an opponent said or did. As parents, we instinctively want to help – to ease their disappointment or frustration and to guide them towards improvement. But too often, our well-meaning advice or attempts to "fix" things can feel overwhelming when all they really want is to be heard.

I've made this mistake more times than I care to admit. I've tried to fast-track my daughter's emotional processing, jumping in with pep talks, constructive criticism, or strategies for next time. But I've come to realise that this isn't what she needs in that moment. What she needs is my quiet support – space to vent, to work through her thoughts, or simply to sit in silence without pressure.

The car ride home is rarely the right time for lessons or solutions. It's a time to listen, to validate, and to remind them that, win or lose, they have our unwavering support. The reflection, the problem-solving, and the plans for improvement can come later, once the emotions have settled and they're ready to talk.

In this chapter, we'll explore how to approach this crucial part of the rugby journey with patience and empathy. How can we create a space where our young players feel supported and understood? How can we show them that, above all else, we value who they are more than how they performed? Let's learn to make the car ride home a moment of connection rather than correction.

1. **"A word of encouragement during a failure is worth more than an hour of praise after success."** – Unknown

2. **"Patience is the companion of wisdom."** – Saint Augustine

3. **"The quieter you become, the more you can hear."** – Ram Dass

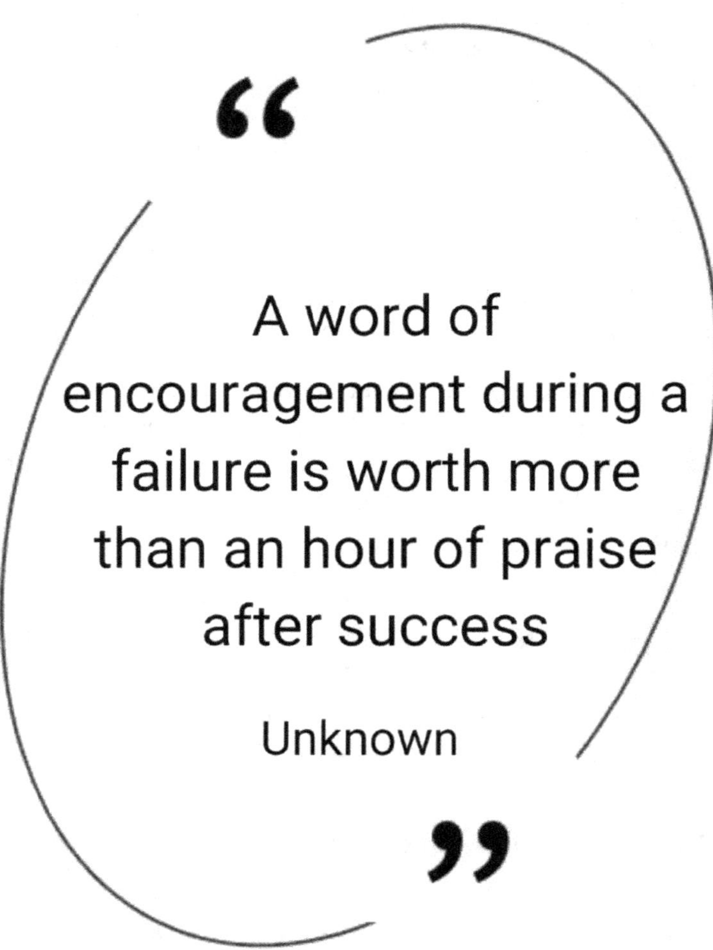

"

A word of
encouragement during a
failure is worth more
than an hour of praise
after success

Unknown

"

Kick-Off: The Quote in Context

As parents, we're quick to praise our children when everything goes right, but this quote challenges us to think differently. When our young rugby player has had a tough game, that's when they need us most – not to dissect what went wrong, but to offer encouragement.

Mistakes and setbacks are inevitable in rugby and in life. They are part of the process of growing, learning, and improving. This quote is a powerful reminder that the support we provide in difficult moments carries far more weight than the congratulations we offer after success. It's in these moments that we can truly make a difference in our child's confidence and resilience.

The Breakdown

In rugby, as in any sport, the match is made up of countless split-second decisions. No one gets every single one right. Even professional players – those at the pinnacle of the sport – make mistakes. Yet, in the heat of competition, it's easy to focus on the errors and forget everything else that went well.

This quote encourages us to flip that narrative. Imagine a young player who has just made a critical mistake – a dropped pass or a missed tackle – that led to the opposition scoring. They're likely already replaying that moment over and over in their mind, feeling embarrassed or frustrated. What they don't need is for us to validate those feelings by pointing out what went wrong.

Instead, they need us to step in with encouragement: to highlight the positive contributions they made, to remind them that everyone makes mistakes, and to help them see the bigger picture. Rugby isn't about perfection; it's about learning and growing through every game, every decision, and yes, every error.

Reflections from Experience

As a parent and coach, I've often found myself in these situations. I remember one particularly challenging match where a young player –

frustrated and teary – came off the pitch after missing several tackles. They sat quietly, avoiding eye contact, clearly replaying those moments in their head.

In that moment, it would have been easy to critique their performance or offer unsolicited advice. Instead, I focused on what went well: their effort in chasing down loose balls, the clever decisions they made under pressure, and their determination to stay involved in the game.

That conversation wasn't about ignoring the mistakes; it was about framing them in a way that helped the player move forward. By the end of the discussion, they had visibly relaxed, and they were smiling again.

I've seen the same dynamic play out with professional players, where fans and commentators zero in on one high-profile mistake, completely overlooking the other 79 minutes of solid play in a particular game. It's a lesson in perspective: no player, at any level, gets it right every time.

Stories from the Sidelines

The sideline can be a high-pressure environment, not just for players but for parents too. It's easy to fall into the trap of critiquing every play or giving unsolicited advice, thinking we're helping. But often, what our children need most on the ride home is our presence and encouragement.

When a game doesn't go as planned, it's a chance to be their anchor. Instead of offering detailed post-match analysis, try reflecting back the effort they put in. Highlight the positives, even if they're small: their commitment to the game, their bravery in trying something new, or their ability to keep going despite setbacks.

Encouragement isn't about pretending mistakes didn't happen; it's about helping our children see mistakes as part of the process. They're not failures – they're opportunities to learn and grow. This shift in mindset helps young players build resilience and confidence, both on and off the pitch.

Half-Time Huddle

1. How do you typically respond when your child has a tough game?

2. Are there ways you can focus on their effort and progress, rather than the outcome?

3. Think about a recent mistake your child made in a game. How could you reframe it as a learning opportunity?

4. How can you balance offering guidance with providing encouragement during challenging moments?

5. What steps can you take to model resilience and a positive attitude toward mistakes in your own life?

Full-Time Whistle

Mistakes are an inevitable part of rugby – and of life. As parents, our role is not to shield our children from these moments but to help them navigate through them. Encouragement in tough times lays the foundation for resilience, confidence, and a lifelong love of the game.

When we focus on effort, progress, and the positives, we teach our children that they are more than their mistakes. We show them that failure is not something to fear but a stepping stone on the path to success.

So, the next time your child comes off the pitch after a challenging game, resist the urge to fix or critique. Instead, offer a kind word, a listening ear, and a reminder of what they did well. It's those moments of encouragement that will stick with them long after the final whistle blows.

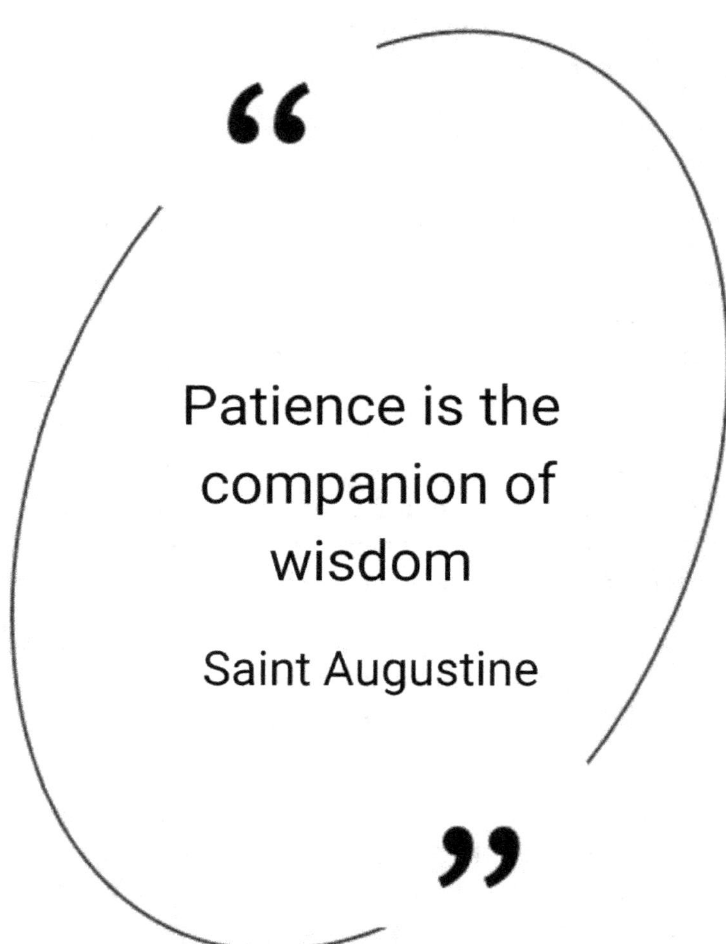
Patience is the companion of wisdom

Saint Augustine

Kick-Off: The Quote in Context

An essential trait that parenting and rugby have in common is the need for patience. Saint Augustine's quote, "Patience is the companion of wisdom," reminds us that wisdom isn't about knowing all the answers but about waiting for the right moment to share them.

For parents of young rugby players, this is particularly relevant. On the journey home after a game, the atmosphere can vary wildly. If the match went well, the conversation flows easily, filled with excitement and pride. But when the game hasn't gone as planned, it's trickier. What do we say? What should we avoid saying? It's in these moments that patience becomes invaluable – not only for our children's growth but for strengthening our relationship with them.

The Breakdown

As parents, it's tempting to jump in with advice. After all, we've lived longer, seen more, and made our fair share of mistakes. But it's important to remember that our experiences, no matter how similar, are not the same as our children's. They process situations in their own unique way, shaped by their age, temperament, and perspective.

Patience allows us to give them the space they need. When a game hasn't gone well, emotions are often running high – frustration, disappointment, or even anger. Rushing in with solutions or unsolicited advice can feel overwhelming or dismissive to them. Instead, waiting until they're ready to talk ensures that when we do share our thoughts, they'll be more receptive.

This approach is especially crucial in rugby, a sport that is both physically and emotionally demanding. Mistakes and setbacks are part of the game, and learning to navigate them requires a level of maturity that takes time to develop. By practising patience, we give our children the opportunity to grow into that maturity at their own pace.

Reflections from Experience

With three daughters playing rugby, I've had plenty of opportunities to learn this lesson the hard way. Each of them processes a tough game differently. One might clam up entirely, another could express her frustrations immediately, while the third has a neutral outward persona that makes it hard to tell what she's feeling.

In the early days, I made the mistake of assuming that a quiet car ride meant an invitation to fill the silence with my analysis of the match. More often than not, this approach backfired. My feedback, no matter how well-intentioned, was met with defensiveness or disinterest.

Over time, I realised that patience was the better approach. By holding back and observing, I began to discern their individual ways of processing emotions. I learned to wait until they were ready to engage, letting them take the lead. Sometimes that meant listening without offering solutions, and other times it meant waiting for them to come to me with questions or concerns.

This shift in approach didn't just improve our post-match conversations; it also deepened our connection. When I gave my daughters the space they needed, they felt respected and supported, which made them more open to my input when the time was right.

Stories from the Sidelines

Patience isn't just for car rides home – it's a skill that's just as important on the sidelines. Every child has their own rhythm when it comes to processing mistakes or tough games. Some bounce back quickly, while others take longer to work through their feelings. As parents, our role is to match their pace, not impose our own.

This might mean letting a young player sit quietly for a while before offering encouragement. It could mean holding back on advice until they ask for it. Or it might mean simply being present, without saying a word, as they sort through their emotions.

In rugby, as in life, patience is a powerful tool. It allows us to step back, observe, and respond thoughtfully rather than react impulsively. And when we model patience for our children, we teach them to approach challenges with the same grace and composure.

Half-Time Huddle

1. How do you typically respond when your child has had a tough game? Could patience play a larger role in those moments?

2. What signals does your child give when they're ready – or not ready – to talk?

3. Are there times when holding back your advice might help your child feel more in control of their emotions and decisions?

4. How can you practise patience not just after the game but during it, as you watch from the sidelines?

5. What lessons about patience can you draw from your own life that might resonate with your young player?

Full-Time Whistle

Patience truly is the companion of wisdom. It's the quiet strength that allows us to wait, observe, and respond in a way that fosters growth and understanding.

For rugby parents, patience means stepping back when emotions are high, giving our children the space to process their experiences, and trusting them to find their way. It means being a steady presence, ready to offer support when they need it but not before.

When we approach parenting with patience, we create an environment where our children feel respected and valued. We teach them that it's okay to take their time, to sit with their emotions, and to find their own solutions. And in doing so, we set them up for success – not just on the rugby pitch but in life.

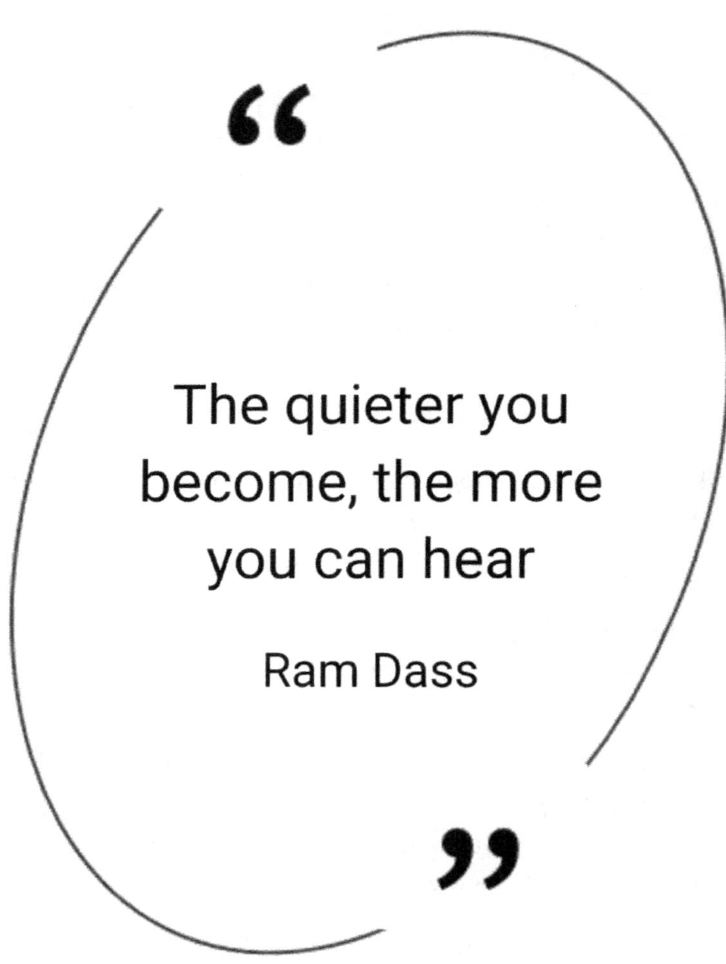
The quieter you
become, the more
you can hear

Ram Dass

Kick-Off: The Quote in Context

"The quieter you become, the more you can hear." These words by Ram Dass resonate deeply with anyone who has taken the time to truly listen – not just with their ears, but with their presence. As parents, particularly those cheering for our kids on the rugby pitch, this quote offers a gentle reminder to pause, step back, and let our young athletes lead the conversation after the game.

It's tempting to rush in with advice or analysis, especially when we're eager to help our children process a tough loss or celebrate a victory. But the car journey home, or any quiet moment after the match, isn't about us setting the agenda. It's about creating space for our children to share their thoughts, feelings, and lessons in their own time.

The Breakdown

In rugby, as in life, listening is a skill that takes patience and practice. It's easy to jump into "fix-it" mode when our children are upset or frustrated after a match. We might offer advice, recount similar experiences, or try to shield them from disappointment. But real growth doesn't happen when we dominate the conversation; it happens when we allow them to navigate their emotions and reflections at their own pace.

Listening isn't just about the words spoken – it's about paying attention to what isn't said. The silences, the body language, the tone of voice – these cues can often tell us more than words ever could. And when we're quiet, when we let the stillness stretch a little longer, we create a safe space where our children can feel heard and supported without pressure.

This doesn't mean ignoring the opportunity to guide them. There will be time to discuss strategies, lessons, or decisions later. But in the immediate aftermath of the game, our job isn't to direct; it's to hold the space for them to process.

Reflections from Experience

I've learned this lesson through years of watching games and riding home in the car with my own children. There have been moments when I've wanted to dive in with advice: "Next time, try to stay in position," or "You could work on tackling lower." But when I held back and listened, I discovered that my children already knew what they needed to work on.

I remember one particular match where my child's team lost by a wide margin. I could see they were upset, and I wanted to say something encouraging right away. Instead, I stayed quiet. After a while, they started talking – about how they felt, what they thought went wrong, and even what they wanted to improve. All I had to do was listen. By the time we reached home, they'd worked through most of their emotions and had a plan for the next practice.

It was a powerful reminder that children often have the answers within them. Our role as parents isn't to give them solutions but to support them as they find their own.

Stories from the Sidelines

Sport is a fantastic testing ground for life skills, and rugby is no exception. It teaches resilience, humility, teamwork, and leadership. But these lessons don't sink in immediately; they unfold over time.

Imagine your child's rugby match as a story. They are the protagonist, navigating challenges and victories. If we, as parents, try to take over the narrative, we rob them of the chance to make the story their own. Instead, we can be the quiet audience, observing and encouraging, so they feel empowered to reflect and learn independently.

True learning is internal. It can't be rushed, and it can't be forced. When we give our children the space to sit with their experiences, they come to their own conclusions – ones that stick with them far longer than any advice we could offer.

Half-Time Huddle

1. Think about the last time your child came to you with a problem. How much space did you give them to express themselves before responding?

2. How can you create an environment where your child feels safe sharing their thoughts after a match?

3. Are there moments when you've rushed to fix or explain a situation, and how might you handle those differently in the future?

4. How can you model patience and active listening for your child, on and off the pitch?

5. What non-verbal cues could you pay more attention to when listening to your child?

Full-Time Whistle

As parents, our natural instinct is to protect, guide, and teach. But sometimes the greatest gift we can offer our children is our silence – the space for them to think, feel, and grow on their own terms.

Rugby is a game, but it's also a microcosm of life. The lessons learned on the pitch – about resilience, teamwork, and leadership – are lessons that will carry our children far beyond the field. By listening without rushing to fix or comment, we show them that their thoughts matter, that we trust their ability to navigate challenges, and that we are there to support them, no matter what.

So next time you're on the drive home from a match, take a breath, stay quiet, and simply listen. You might be surprised at what you hear.

Chapter 4

Once the Mud Has Dried

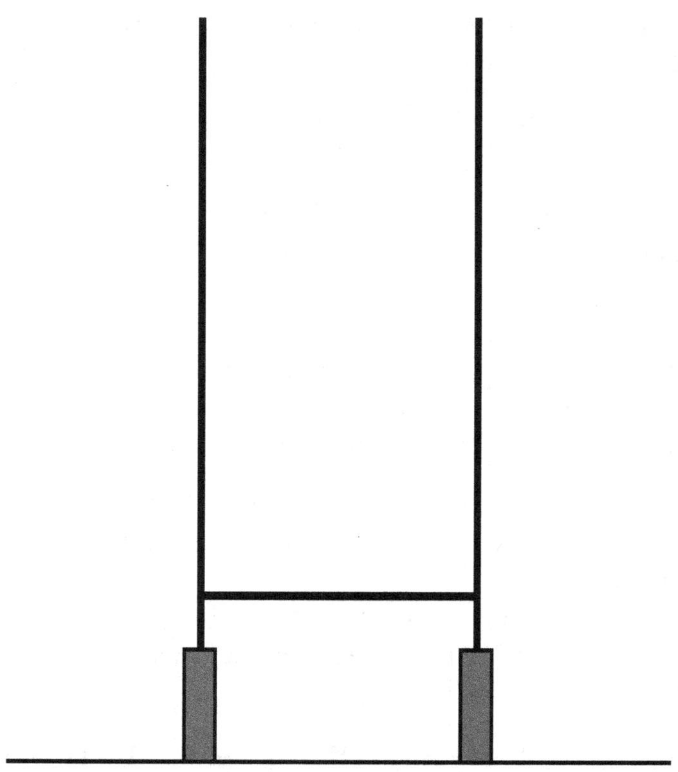

A day or two after the game or training session, once the boots are cleaned (or at least out of the car) and the mud has dried, we enter a different phase of reflection. The intensity of the moment has passed, and emotions have had time to settle. It's in this calmer space that meaningful conversations can take place – ones that help our young players make sense of their experience and grow from it.

This is the time to truly listen, to understand their perspective without the haze of immediate frustration or excitement clouding the discussion. Perhaps they've gained clarity on what went well or what didn't, and as parents, we can offer our observations in a way that complements theirs. By focusing on connection and curiosity, we can encourage them to take valuable lessons from the experience, without it feeling like criticism or pressure.

It's still vital to ensure that our young players feel heard. This isn't about lecturing or telling them how they *should* feel, but about creating a space where they can reflect with openness. When they're ready, we can guide the conversation towards constructive insights – helping them see how to build on their strengths and approach challenges with confidence.

In this final chapter, we'll explore how to make the most of this reflective time. How can we nurture their growth, resilience, and love for the game? How can we use this window of calm to reinforce the values that sport – and life – teaches? Once the mud has dried, let's help our children see the bigger picture and take their next steps with positivity and purpose.

1. **"Most people do not listen with the intent to understand; they listen with the intent to reply."** – *Stephen R. Covey*

2. ***"The greatest glory in living lies not in never falling, but in rising every time we fall."*** – *Nelson Mandela*

3. **"Fix It."** – *Patrick Hickman*

"

Most people do not
listen with the intent
to understand; they
listen with the intent
to reply

Stephen R. Covey

"

Kick-Off: The Quote in Context

Stephen Covey's insight on listening hits home for many of us, especially as parents. It's all too easy to fall into the habit of listening just long enough to jump in with advice, an answer, or a "teachable moment." But Covey reminds us to pause and truly understand – not just the words, but the feelings, thoughts, and experiences being shared.

As rugby parents, we have a unique opportunity to create meaningful connections with our children through this kind of listening. Whether it's after a match or in the quiet days that follow, the way we listen can shape not only their understanding of the game but also their ability to navigate life's ups and downs.

The Breakdown

Listening to understand requires us to put aside our urge to fix or teach and instead focus on what our child is truly saying – or not saying. After a match, it might be tempting to jump straight into analysis: "Why didn't you pass sooner?" or "You could work on not bunching up around the ball." But if we listen with curiosity and patience, we may discover that their focus is elsewhere.

Younger players might be bursting with excitement, eager to recount every play, while older children might be quieter, reflecting internally on what went well and what didn't. Their way of processing can change over time, and part of our job is to adjust our approach to meet them where they are.

Understanding their world requires asking thoughtful questions and being genuinely curious. It's not about prying but about creating a space where they feel safe to share. The more we show that we understand their perspective – or at least acknowledge the challenges they face – the more receptive they'll be to any guidance we might offer later.

Reflections from Experience

I've learned that the way I listen to my children after a match makes all the difference. There have been times when I thought I was helping by giving immediate feedback, only to realise I'd completely missed the mark. One time after a particularly tough game, I started pointing out areas for improvement, thinking I was being constructive. My child, clearly frustrated, eventually said, "I already know what I did wrong – I just wanted you to listen."

It was a wake-up call. From then on, I made a conscious effort to approach these conversations differently. Instead of diving in with advice, I started asking open-ended questions like, "How do you think the game went?" or "What was the best part for you?" More often than not, they already had the answers or were working through their own reflections. My role wasn't to provide solutions – it was to support them in finding their own.

Stories from the Sidelines

Rugby offers countless opportunities for learning, but those lessons don't always emerge immediately. John Dewey's words, "We do not learn from experience; we learn from reflecting on experience," hold true here. Reflection takes time, and every child processes at their own pace.

Younger players might chatter endlessly about their match, eager to relive the highs and lows, while teenagers might need more space and silence before they're ready to talk. As parents, it's up to us to recognise these differences and adapt our approach.

For example, if your child is quiet after a match, resist the urge to fill the silence. Instead, let them take the lead. When they're ready, they'll share what's on their mind. And when they do, show them that you're listening – not just hearing the words but truly understanding their feelings and experiences.

When your child feels understood, they're more likely to be open to your guidance. But remember, timing is everything. Even the best advice won't land if it's delivered when they're not ready to hear it.

Half-Time Huddle

1. Reflect on how you usually respond after a match. Do you listen to understand, or do you focus on offering advice?

2. How well do you adapt your approach to your child's age and personality?

3. What questions could you ask to encourage your child to share their thoughts and feelings?

4. Can you recall a time when your advice was well-received? What made that moment different?

5. How can you create a safe and supportive environment for your child to reflect and learn?

Full-Time Whistle

Listening is an art, and as parents, it's one of the most powerful tools we have. By listening with the intent to understand, we show our children that their feelings and experiences matter.

Rugby teaches many things such as discipline, adaptability, and problem-solving, but these lessons take time to unfold. As parents, our role is to create the conditions for learning – not by providing all the answers but by supporting our children as they discover their own.

Next time you feel the urge to offer advice after a match, take a moment, stay present, and listen with the intention of understanding what your child has to say. You might find that what your child needs most isn't your words but your presence and understanding.

"

The greatest glory in living lies not in never falling, but in rising every time we fall

Nelson Mandela

"

Kick-Off: The Quote in Context

Nelson Mandela's words carry a timeless message: life's greatest triumphs come not from avoiding failure but from how we respond to it. It's an idea that resonates deeply with rugby, a sport where resilience is tested with every tackle, fumble, and setback.

As parents, we're uniquely positioned to help our children navigate these challenges. Rugby isn't just about the scores or the trophies – it's about the lessons learned through both victory and defeat. By teaching our children how to rise after a fall, we help them develop resilience that extends far beyond the pitch.

The Breakdown

Falling is inevitable in rugby, just as it is in life. A missed pass, a dropped ball, or a lost match can feel monumental in the heat of the moment. But these moments are not the end – they're stepping stones to growth.

In rugby, the next job is always waiting. The referee hasn't blown the whistle, so the game goes on. It's this mindset – moving forward, tackling the next challenge – that builds character. Teaching our children to approach life this way helps them see setbacks as temporary and surmountable.

We can also help them view their mistakes in context. A single error doesn't define a match, just as a single failure doesn't define a person. When the dust settles, our role is to provide perspective and support, helping them see the bigger picture and find the lessons within.

Reflections from Experience

I've seen this lesson play out countless times. One match stands out where my child made a critical mistake, leading to a try for the opposition. At the final whistle, their disappointment was palpable. On the car ride home, I wanted to jump in with reassurances and advice, but instead, I just listened.

Later that evening, they came to me, still upset but ready to talk. We discussed the match, and they began to see not just the mistake but also the moments where they had played well. By the end of the conversation, their frustration had turned into determination to train harder and improve.

Moments like these remind me that the greatest gift we can give our children is not solving their problems but equipping them with the resilience to face them head-on.

Stories from the Sidelines

Rugby provides endless examples of resilience. A young player might drop the ball but sprint back to make a tackle moments later. A team may be down by several tries yet claw their way back through sheer grit and teamwork.

These are the stories that inspire us, but they're not just for the players on the pitch – they're for us as parents, too. Don't be afraid to let your children see you stumble. Whether it's an error at work or a moment of frustration, showing them how you recover demonstrates resilience in action.

When they see you get back up, they learn that failure isn't something to fear. It's a natural part of life and an opportunity to grow stronger. By modelling this behaviour, you give them permission to do the same.

Half-Time Huddle

1. How do you react when your child faces challenges on or off the pitch? Are you quick to offer solutions, or do you take time to listen?

2. What lessons have you learned from your own mistakes, and how can you share these with your child?

3. How do you help your child process setbacks and see the bigger picture?

4. Think about a time when you demonstrated resilience to your child – how did they respond?

5. How can you encourage your child to focus on "the next job" instead of dwelling on setbacks?

Full-Time Whistle

Resilience is a skill that's built over time, one stumble at a time. By helping our children embrace their falls and focus on getting back up, we prepare them for the challenges they'll face in life.

Mandela's words remind us that true glory lies not in avoiding failure but in rising again. As rugby parents, we have the privilege of guiding our children through this process, both on and off the pitch.

So, let's celebrate the stumbles, the scrapes, and the muddy jerseys. Each fall is an opportunity to rise stronger, to learn, and to grow. And when we rise alongside them, we remind them – and ourselves – that the game isn't over until the final whistle blows.

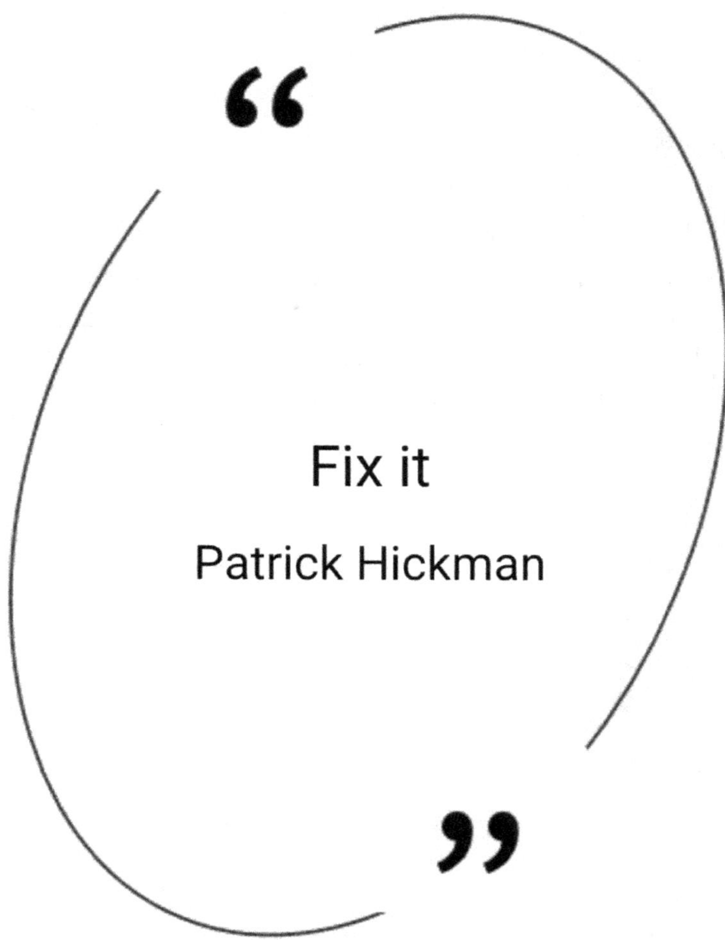

Fix it

Patrick Hickman

Kick-Off: The Quote in Context

"Fix it." Two simple words, but they carry the weight of resilience, accountability, and forward momentum. These words often leave my lips when I'm coaching or watching a rugby match – whether it's one of my daughters' teams, or any other of our club's teams. The inspiration behind this mantra struck me whilst watching one of our Women's 1stXV matches. As I watched the players navigate the game's ups and downs, it hit me: this is what rugby – and life – is all about.

In rugby, mistakes are inevitable. A dropped ball, a missed tackle, or a botched pass – these moments happen to everyone. But what separates an average player from a great one is what happens next. The game doesn't stop when something goes wrong. You can't go back, but you can always move forward. And this truth extends far beyond the pitch.

The Breakdown

Mistakes are a universal experience, both in rugby and in life. In the heat of a match, the temptation to dwell on a blunder can be overwhelming. Frustration might take over, or embarrassment might creep in, paralysing the player from taking the next step. But there's no time for wallowing.

In rugby, as in life, the game doesn't stop until the referee blows the whistle. Until then, you have an opportunity – a chance to fix it. The question isn't whether you'll mess up; it's what you'll do about it.

"Fix it" is about action. If you've knocked on the ball, your next job is to secure possession or realign the defence. Missed a tackle? Sprint back and help recover. It's about looking forward, not back. The beauty of rugby is that it teaches us this lesson over and over again. Life, similarly, gives us countless chances to course correct.

Reflections from Experience

I've said "fix it" more times than I can count, whether on the sideline or at home. As a coach and a parent, I've seen firsthand how this mindset transforms not only games but also attitudes. One moment that stands out was when my youngest daughter, after missing a critical tackle, momentarily froze on the pitch. I could see the frustration in her body language. But then, something shifted. She shook it off, sprinted back, and disrupted the opposing team's play. That single act of resilience turned the game around.

The same principle applies to everyday life. Mistakes happen – a missed opportunity at work, a misunderstanding with a friend, or a moment of poor judgment. Like on the pitch, you have two choices: let the mistake define you or take action to correct it. I've learned that showing my daughters this philosophy in my own life – rather than just saying it – is what truly cements its value. Whether it's owning up to an error at work or making amends for a misstep in a relationship, the lesson is clear: fix it and move on.

Stories from the Sidelines

In rugby, fixing it isn't always about heroics. Often, it's about the small, unglamorous actions that contribute to the team's success. A dropped ball doesn't need a miracle; it needs a quick dive to secure possession. A missed kick isn't the end of the match; it's a call to focus on the next phase.

Similarly, life's challenges rarely require grand gestures. Most often, they demand humility and a willingness to try again. Whether it's apologising after a mistake or reevaluating a failed plan, fixing it is a step-by-step process. The key is to keep moving, no matter how small the steps may seem.

Half-Time Huddle

1. Think about a recent mistake or setback. How did you respond? Could you have focused more on fixing it rather than dwelling on it?

2. How can you teach your young rugby player – or yourself – that a mistake isn't the end but an opportunity to grow?

3. What small, practical steps can you take the next time something goes wrong to ensure you're moving forward?

4. How can the "fix it" philosophy strengthen teamwork, both on and off the pitch?

5. What role does resilience play in helping us recover from mistakes and find the next opportunity to succeed?

Full-Time Whistle

"Fix it" is a call to action, a reminder that mistakes are inevitable but not final. In rugby, it's about doing the next job, helping your team recover, and keeping the game moving. In life, it's about taking responsibility, finding solutions, and learning from each experience.

Whether you're coaching, playing, or simply navigating the complexities of daily life, this mindset is transformative. It shifts the focus from what's gone wrong to what can still go right. So, the next time you – or your child – faces a setback, remember: the game isn't over. Fix it and keep going.

Wrap Up

As we wrap up this book, I want to thank you for joining me in exploring the unique and rewarding journey of being a rugby parent. The insights shared here are simply what I've discovered along the way, shaped by my own experiences and reflections. They're not definitive answers but rather an invitation to think about what works best for you and your family.

I hope the reflective questions throughout have offered you moments of clarity and helped you uncover your own ways to navigate the ups and downs of this adventure. Whether it's finding calm in pre-match tensions, staying grounded during the game, or creating space for post-match emotions, the aim has always been to make the journey a little smoother and more enjoyable – for both you and your young player.

I'm not the finished article, and none of us are. This journey, much like rugby itself, is about growth – learning as we go and supporting our young players as they embrace the game we all love. Rugby, like parenting, is filled with moments of learning, connection, and joy. I hope this book has added something meaningful to your experience.

Thank you for allowing me to share my thoughts with you – here's to many more muddy, joyful memories ahead.

References for Quotes Used in This Book

1. "It's not what you look at that matters, it's what you see." – Henry David Thoreau
   From *Walden and Other Writings* (1854).

2. "Doubt kills more dreams than failure ever will." – Suzy Kassem
   From *Rise Up and Salute the Sun* (2011).

3. "It's not the load that breaks you down; it's the way you carry it."
   – Lou Holtz
   Widely attributed in sports commentary, exact source uncertain.

4. "Sometimes the most important thing in a whole day is the rest we take between two deep breaths." – Etty Hillesum
   From *An Interrupted Life: The Diaries, 1941–1943* (1983).

5. "Correction does much, but encouragement does more." – Johann Wolfgang von Goethe
   From *Maxims and Reflections* (1821).

6. "I've failed over and over and over again in my life. And that is why I succeed." – Michael Jordan
   Quoted in *For the Love of the Game: My Story* (1998).

7. "A word of encouragement during a failure is worth more than an hour of praise after success." – Unknown
   Commonly cited in motivational works, original source unclear.

8. "Patience is the companion of wisdom." – Saint Augustine
   From *The Confessions of Saint Augustine* (circa 400 CE).

9. "The quieter you become, the more you can hear." – Ram Dass
   From *Be Here Now* (1971).

10. "Most people do not listen with the intent to understand; they listen with the intent to reply." – Stephen R. Covey
    From *The 7 Habits of Highly Effective People* (1989).

11. "The greatest glory in living lies not in never falling, but in rising every time we fall." – Nelson Mandela
From *Long Walk to Freedom: The Autobiography of Nelson Mandela* (1994).

12. "Fix It." – Patrick Hickman
Original insight by the author.